T0252864

Thieme

Plates for
Color Vision Testing

Joern Kuchenbecker, MD
Head of Eye Clinic
HELIOS Hospital Berlin-Buch
Berlin, Germany

Dieter Broschmann, MD
Professor Emeritus of Ophthalmology
Berlin, Germany

Founded and advanced by
Jakob Stilling
Ernst Hertel
Karl Velhagen

32 illustrations

Georg Thieme Verlag
Stuttgart · New York

Library of Congress Cataloging-in-Publication Data is available from the publisher.

This book is an authorized translation of the 34th German edition published and copyrighted 2011 by Georg Thieme Verlag, Stuttgart. Title of the German edition: Tafeln zur Prüfung des Farbsinnes

Translator: Gertrud Champe, Surry, Maine, USA

© 2014 Georg Thieme Verlag KG,
Rüdigerstrasse 14, 70469 Stuttgart, Germany
http://www.thieme.de
Thieme Medical Publishers, Inc.,
333 Seventh Avenue,
New York, NY 10001, USA
http://www.thieme.com

Cover design: Thieme Publishing Group
Typesetting by primustype Robert Hurler GmbH, Notzingen, Germany
Printed in Germany by Karl Grammlich GmbH, Pliezhausen, Germany

ISBN 978-313-175481-3

Foreword

The pseudoisochromatic color plates first created by Stilling and further developed by Hertel, Velhagen, and Broschmann, have been published by Thieme Publishers for over a hundred years. Fortunately, an English language version of these plates is now available.

This edition consists of 32 color plates for screening of red-green and blue-yellow deficiencies. The color plates used to screen for blue-yellow deficiencies are placed at the end of the test series because these deficiencies are relatively rare. The plates to screen for red-green deficiencies include some color plates that were already used by Stilling and Hertel.

The color plates are based on the premise that the *subject* does not know the number and kind of characters (Arabic numerals and Latin letters) to be read on each plate. For children, dyslexic patients, and illiterate patients, there are several plates with tumbling E's so that a large range of individuals can be tested for color vision.

Joern Kuchenbecker, MD

1 Notes on the Use of the Plates

Explanation

The plates are intended to make it possible for ophthalmologists, practitioners of general and occupational medicine or other specialties, and also medical assistants, teachers, artists, technologists, and other interested non-physicians to make a very probable assessment of an individual's color vision. A procedure of this sort cannot be completely free of error. Therefore, the objective must be to arrive at fewer false positives than false negatives, which can then be corrected with another method. The plates should be usable for routine medical screening, that is, the time required should be reasonable. Therefore, it has been necessary to limit their number.

Physiological Premises

The following explanations are offered to clarify the understanding of the physiology and pathology of color vision.

Normally, human color vision can distinguish about 200 different color shades, about 26 degrees of saturation and about 500 different degrees of intensity (Erb and Fahle 2006) and no language has the words for anywhere near the number of corresponding names. Technology uses special classification systems, such as CIELAB or CIELUV.

The receptors on which human color vision is based comprise **three types of cones** whose outer segments are filled with a short (**cyanolabe**), a medium (**chlorolabe**), and a long-wavelength-sensitive photopigment (**erythrolabe**). These are the components of all those characteristics of color vision that are called "**trichromatic**" (Boynton 1988, Conway 2009, De Valois and Abramov 1966, Gegenfurtner and Kiper 2003, Jacobs 1976, Krastel 1995, Lanthony 1987, Lennie and D'Zmura 1988, Michael 1973, Nathans 1999, Ripps and Weale 1969, Swanson and Cohen 2003, Walraven 1972).

It is insufficient to explain color vision on the basis of the receptors alone. The attempt to do this led to a historical controversy between the adherents of Young (1802) and Helmholtz (1867, 1892) who saw clear evidence for a trichromatic structure of color vision, and the adherents of Hering (1874) on the other hand, who had equally good arguments for a **color antagonistic** structure.

Kries formulated a synthesis of the two theories in 1897 in his **zone theory**, which has been experimentally confirmed (Krastel 1995). The zone theory states that physical color stimuli impinging on the retina are received as described by the three-color theory while their neuronal transmission to the brain proceeds as described in the color-antagonistic theory (Welsch and Liebmann 2003).

Anomalies in color vision are colloquially known as "color blindness" or "color deficiency." The preferred terminology is to call individuals with normal color vision **color-normal** and those with abnormal color vision **color-anomalous** or **color-deficient**.

Congenital Disorders

Classification

With few exceptions, congenital disorders can be organized into a single scheme. The following types are identified:

Monochromatism (Achromatopsia, Total Color Blindness)
A person with monochromatic vision only sees variations between black and white, comparable to black and white photography. Colors are not experienced as such but appear as shades of gray.

Dichromatism (Two-color Vision)
Lay persons usually describe this deficiency inexactly and superficially as "color blindness." The affected individual experiences only two color groups. The disorder appears in three color variants, designated by Greek number names according to the color's position in the spectrum:
- Protanopia ("red blindness")
- Deuteranopia ("green blindness")
- Tritanopia ("blue blindness")

The color experience of affected individuals is limited to variants of two colors and to variations of black and white as shades of gray.

Because of the unfortunate expression "color blindness," the lay person often imagines that a person with red or green blindness cannot see colored objects, that is, that the person is "blind" to them. This occurs only very rarely, for example, with a very muted dark red (e.g., dirty rear lights of a car). A person with anomalous color vision also sees colored objects, but as being of a color different from what the color-normal person sees. Confusions occur, such as with traffic lights, ripe and unripe strawberries, and fabrics. The affected person knows that blood is red and not green and that an agitated person turns red and not green, that the sun is red when it sets and grass is green. And often, there are secondary hints and clues for such a person. He or she knows that on traffic signals, the red light is at the top, the green light is at the bottom, and the yellow light is in the middle. But as soon as the color appears out of context, the individual with anomalous color vision becomes insecure and makes mistakes.

Anomalous Trichromatism (Anomalous Three-color Vision)
Numerous colors from all regions of the spectrum are experienced but one of the three components is under-represented. To have the same color experience from a mixed color as a color-normal person, the individual with trichromatism must add more of the color for which his or her color vision is deficient. To a color-normal person, the result of such a mixture appears to be affected with a color cast.
Subgroups of anomalous trichromatism are:
- Protanomaly ("red deficiency")
- Deuteranomaly ("green deficiency")
- Tritanomaly ("blue deficiency")

Since the boundaries between the color-vision deficiencies are not sharply delimited and have little practical significance, the terms for individuals with dichromatism and congenital anomalous trichromatism are combined as follows:
- Protanopia and protanomaly = **Protans**
- Deuteranopia and deuteranomaly = **Deuterans**
- Tritanopia and tritanomaly = **Tritans**

Epidemiology and Inheritance

In Western Europe, hereditary, X-chromosome recessive **red-green deficiency** is found in approximately 8% of men and only 0.4 to 0.5% of women, while 15% of women are heterozygous carriers (Deeb and Motulsky 2005, Krastel 1995). Approximately 3% of Black African men and 4 to 6% of Japanese and Chinese men exhibit color deficiency. The frequency of the individual types of color deficiency varies. In the male population of Western Europe, 5% are deuteranomalous and 1% are protanomalous, protanopes, and deuteranopes respectively (Deeb and Motulsky 2005, Krastel 1995).

In numbers and actual practice, there are only a very few **congenital tritans** (order of magnitude 1:10,000 to 1:60,000; Kalmus 1955). They have a gene mutation on chromosome 7 that codes for the blue cone pigment (cyanolabe) (Weitz et al 1992a, 1992b). Inheritance is autosomal dominant, and expression is correspondingly variable (Krastel 1995).

Inheritance of **congenital achromatopsia** (congenital total color blindness or rod **monochromatism**) is autosomal recessive. Incidence of the complete form is estimated to be approximately 1:30,000 (Krastel 1995, Zrenner 1985). Mutations in CNGA3 (chromosome 2), CNGB3 (chromosome 8) and GNAT2 (chromosome 1) are responsible (Deeb and Motulsky 2005). Monochromats are usually already recognized because of other anomalies such as poor visual acuity, involuntary eye movements (nystagmus), photophobia, and albinism among others.

Thus, in practice, almost only protans and deuterans need to be diagnosed.

Acquired Disorders

Acquired disorders of color vision cannot always be forced into this scheme since they include all the steps between good vision and blindness. As processes or their consequences, they can either progress or improve. They can be important for the recognition of certain diseases or types of poisoning; under certain circumstances they only affect parts of the visual field. As a rule, it is not these but other visual disorders that motivate the patient to consult a physician. Sometimes they cause the environment to appear in a certain color, for instance yellow with certain anthelminthics and red with digitalis glycosides. For all people, color sense depends on certain external and internal conditions. These are qualities of the colors themselves, such as hue, brightness, and saturation, as well as the condition of the visual organs, such as light–dark adaptation, and prior color impressions, color of the surroundings, size of the colored object, and duration of the visual exposure.

Functional Principle of the Plates

The technical principle used in most examination plates is the principle discovered by Donders and introduced by Stilling of so-called **pseudoisochromasia**: on a colored background pattern numbers or letters are drawn in. They differ from the background by color but not by brightness. Since the individual with deficient color vision does not recognize the color, he or she cannot distinguish the background from the digits represented at the same brightness and thus cannot read them (**Plates 4–10, 12–17**).

In some **plates**, the principle of pseudoisochromasia is combined with the opposite principle of pseudoanisochromasia. On a colored background pattern with numbers or letters of different colors, additional numbers or letters of a different brightness are drawn in. The color differences are very clear to a color-normal person; for a color-deficient person, only the brightness differences are noticeable (**Plates 2, 3, 11**).

2 Instructions for Use

General Points

- Never touch the plates or allow them to be touched.
- Do not expose to light unnecessarily.
- Never store in a damp or hot environment.
- Do not hand the plates to the test subject.

The plates must not be allowed to become marked by spots, wrinkles, and certainly not pencil marks. For the examiner's convenience, there are small, inverted numbers in the margin. Care must be taken that other test subjects present, in the case of large-scale screening, do not see the plates or hear the answers of the subjects being tested before them (they may learn the answers or the order by heart). The plates are displayed at approximately 70-cm intervals. Avoid direct sunlight on the plates. In all pigment color tests, such as the pseudoisochromatic plates, correct illumination is integral to the examination because pigment colors only reflect the light with which they are illuminated (Erb et al 1999, Hardy et al, 1946, Krastel 1995, Krastel et al 2009, Volk and Fry 1947). The intensity of the light should be 400 to 1,000 lux of white light. Appropriate white light sources are bulbs with continuous, daylight-like emission for color sampling. The correlated color temperature should be above 5,000 to 6,800 K (Krastel 2007).

Subjects must not be allowed to read at an angle, at variable distances, or with back and forth movements. They may only see the plate for 15 seconds. Usually, distance glasses may be worn for the test. The examination is conducted for both eyes, one eye at a time, since the results can differ, both in congenital and acquired color-vision deficiency.

Administering the Test

Subjects who can read Arabic numbers and Latin letters are first shown **Plate 1**, which any individual with a color defect can recognize. Explain that there are one to three characters on each plate, either letters or numbers.

Children, subjects who have difficulty reading, or those who are illiterate are first shown **Plates 18 and 19**. The examiner explains that the subject should show the opening of the "trident." This can be done either with a trident that is held as on the plate or by telling or showing the direction of the trident by drawing it in the air the way it is on the plate, without touching the paper. Subjects who do not understand this task or cannot carry it out may also be shown **Plate 29**. Here, the subject must show the course of the line in the air. This general explanation can be given to a large group of test subjects from a greater distance. Then the other plates are displayed in order. If you suspect that a test subject has learned the plates by heart, change the order and repeat individual plates. In the case of the trident, the book can be turned, so as to change the direction. In the log, mark "right," "wrong," or "not read." The final evaluation can be "pass," "fail," or "uncertain."

Table 2.1 gives an overview of **Plates 1–32** with correct answers.

Table 2.1 Overview of the plates

Plate No.	Answer: Color-normal	Answer: Color-deficient	Description
1	2L	2L	Demonstration plate
2	182	Red-green deficiency: 8 Blue-yellow deficiency: 12	Diagnostic plate
3	69	Red-green deficiency: 60, 66, 00	Transformation plate
4	25	Red-green deficiency: no answer or wrong answer	Vanishing plate
5	3	Red-green deficiency: no answer or wrong answer	Vanishing plate
6	6R	Red-green deficiency: no answer or wrong answer	Vanishing plate
7	2	Red-green deficiency: no answer or wrong answer	Vanishing plate
8	F4	Red-green deficiency: no answer or wrong answer	Vanishing plate
9	6	Red-green deficiency: no answer or wrong answer	Vanishing plate
10	51	Red-green deficiency: no answer or wrong answer	Vanishing plate
11	3	Red-green deficiency: 8	Transformation plate
12	94	Red-green deficiency: no answer or wrong answer	Vanishing plate

Table 2.1 Overview of the plates (cont.)

Plate No.	Answer: Color-normal	Answer: Color-deficient	Description
13	42	Red-green deficiency: no answer or wrong answer	Vanishing plate
14	65	Red-green deficiency: no answer or wrong answer	Vanishing plate
15	RG	Red-green deficiency: no answer or wrong answer	Vanishing plate
16	A4	Red-green deficiency: no answer or wrong answer	Vanishing plate
17	68	Red-green deficiency: no answer or wrong answer	Vanishing plate
18	Trident (right open)	Only malingerers give wrong answer	Demonstration plate
19	Trident (left open)	Only malingerers give wrong answer	Demonstration plate
20	Trident (top open)	Red-green deficiency: no answer or wrong answer	Vanishing plate
21	Trident (right open)	Red-green deficiency: no answer or wrong answer	Vanishing plate
22	Trident bottom open)	Red-green deficiency: no answer or wrong answer	Vanishing plate
23	Trident (left open)	Red-green deficiency: no answer or wrong answer	Vanishing plate
24	Trident (right open)	Red-green deficiency: no answer or wrong answer	Vanishing plate
25	Trident (top open)	Red-green deficiency: no answer or wrong answer	Vanishing plate
26	Trident (right open)	Red-green deficiency: no answer or wrong answer	Vanishing plate
27	Trident (left open)	Red-green deficiency: no answer or wrong answer	Vanishing plate
28	Trident (bottom open)	Red-green deficiency: no answer or wrong answer	Vanishing plate
29	Line can be followed	Red-green deficiency: line cannot be followed	Vanishing plate
30	49	Blue-yellow deficiency: no answer or wrong answer	Vanishing plate
31	5E	Blue-yellow deficiency: no answer or wrong answer	Vanishing plate
32	45	Blue-yellow deficiency: no answer or wrong answer	Vanishing plate

Agitated, anxious test subjects sometimes do not dare to name the characters because they feel unsure. The subjects should be encouraged and, if necessary, be allowed to draw the signs in the air with an index finger or a reversed pencil (without touching the paper!). After this, the examination often proceeds quite easily.

Shortening or Simplifying the Examination Process

This is always questionable. **Under no circumstances** is it permitted to shorten the examination. The test has only been passed if all plates have been correctly described. If appropriate, a reading error can be corrected.

3 Diagnosis

Doubtful Cases

The evaluation "color-vision doubtful" cannot always be avoided with pigment color tests. Agitated and anxious patients have already been mentioned. Tracing the signs in the air is almost always possible. There are a small number of individuals who are not of an intelligence level capable of going through any test. Colloquially, they are called "color ignorant." But even they can often trace out the characters. It is better to evaluate a test subject as doubtful and refer him or her for additional examination than simply guess whether he or she is color-normal, since professional development may depend on the diagnosis. The doubtful cases may include acquired disorders associated with various diseases and types of poisoning. An examination can be evaluated as passed if the subject's only error is to read 66 instead of 6R (**Plate 6**) but correct it on second reading, or if he or she only reads the two numbers at the edges of **Plate 2** after being prompted. The ophthalmologist may also have a choice of further collections of plates and tests:
* The Ishihara color plates
* The Farnsworth-Munsell 100 hue test
* The lantern test (Lanthony panel D15 test or other)
* Anomaloscope
Usually the ophthalmologist will be able to recognize acquired disorders by means of a complete eye examination.
The following cases **must be referred for additional examinations**:
* The test subject cannot be convinced of the examination results.
* The subject passes the plate examination but fails in daily practice.
* The simulation or dissimulation question (see below) was not clarified.
* Suspicion of blue-yellow disorder.
* Suspicion of complete color blindness.

- Increased occupational responsibility, for example, in traffic management, the textile industry, referrals of physicians and persons who must themselves conduct examinations with the plates.
- If only one or two slight errors were made but the subject hesitated, blinked, shaded their eyes, moved their head back and forth, and/or needed a particularly long time.
- Forensic cases.

Simulation and Dissimulation

Simulation: In liability and criminal proceedings or if it seems useful to the subject for other reasons to pretend that he or she is color-vision-deficient, there is a risk of simulation. A test subject excites suspicion if they claim that they cannot recognize **Plates 1, 18, and 19**. It is equally suspicious if no colors at all are recognized where no eye defects exist.

Dissimulation: An interest in concealing a color-vision deficiency exists among applicants for certain occupations, for example, traffic management, for which normal color vision or only slightly limited color vision is required. They try to obtain the plates in order to learn them by heart. Tracing out the characters in the air and correct reading of the plates is impossible for them if the order of the plates is changed.

Differential Diagnosis

An experienced examiner is very likely to be able to establish a differential diagnosis of the individual forms of color-vision disorders, especially when the protan fails noticeably in tests with dark red on dark green. The failure rate, however, is too high to base an important differentiation on this test alone.

It is quite possible to distinguish "mild" and "severe" disorders on the basis of the error score, but it is never possible to guarantee that the subject with a "mild color-vision deficiency" might not fail in an individual case under some accidentally very unfavorable conditions (small object, short viewing time, poor lighting, glare, colored surroundings, contrast, etc.). Tritans fail with **Plates 2 and 30–32**, for example.

However, it is not the case that each group only reads certain plates confidently and without error. There are many plates on which both protans and deuterans fail.

4 Counseling the Examinees

At present, we are not able to cure, improve, or eliminate by exercise a congenital color-vision deficiency in human beings. The color names of certain objects can be learned (e.g., the colors of national flags, fire trucks, and so on), but this does not allow the color-deficient individual to experience the color as the color-normal individual does.

A certain **practical aid** that is very seldom used are **colored monocular filter lenses**, one red and one green. Green objects appear brighter through a green lens and redder through a red lens, whereas objects of other colors seem darker. Colored glasses sold as sunglasses or protective glasses can possibly have similar effects but in fact they may lead to new errors.

Many individuals with color-vision deficiencies correctly point out that in practice they have so far never failed. This is due to the fact that there are numerous secondary assistive devices that aid in recognition of the object. Drivers of vehicles and all participants in traffic must know that they must never rely on the signal color alone and that in case of a moving violation they cannot use color-vision deficiency, of which they were aware, as an excuse. Protans are especially at risk of late recognition of rear and brake lights, particularly under foggy conditions (Cole 2002).

With regard to requirements for color vision in various occupations, it is necessary to consult the regulations of individual countries, since they often vary from one country to another and are often changed.

Physicians can recognize low-grade or chronic poisoning due to long-term use or misuse of medicines (antirheumatics, sedatives, hypnotics, appetite depressants), of nicotine and alcohol, and exposure to chemical noxae (e.g., lead) on the basis of color-vision deficiencies. Deficiencies in color vision can be an early symptom in chronic liver diseases. Serious evaluation problems can result when a person with deficient color vision ascribes a previously unrecognized congenital color-vision deficiency to a prescription medicine.

5 Self-examination by the Examiner

It is essential for all examiners to be examined themselves. If they cannot read the plates themselves they are inclined to believe that this is simply impossible, instead of mistrusting their own color vision.

References

Boynton RM. Color vision. Annu Rev Psychol 1988; 39: 69–100

Cole BL. Protan colour vision deficiency and road accidents. Clin Exp Optom 2002; 85: 246–253

Conway BR. Color vision, cones, and color-coding in the cortex. Neuroscientist 2009; 15: 274–290

De Valois RL, Abramov I. Color vision. Annu Rev Psychol 1966; 17: 337–362

Deeb SS, Motulsky AG. Red-Green Color Vision Defects. In: RA Pagon, TC Bird, CR Dolan, K Stephens, eds. GeneReviews. Seattle: National Center for Biotechnology Information; 2005

Erb C, Fahle M. Farbensehen und erworbene Farbsinnstörungen. Teil I: Grundlagen. Ophthalmologe 2006; 103: 349–360

Erb C, Ulrich A, Adler M, et al. Influence of illumination on results of the hue-discrimination test, Roth 28-Hue desaturated. Neuro-ophthalmology 1999; 22: 33–36

Gegenfurtner KR, Kiper DC. Color vision. Annu Rev Neurosci 2003; 26: 181–206

Hardy LH, Rand G, Rittler MC. Effect of quality of illumination on the results of the Ishihara test. Arch Ophthal 1946; 36: 685–699

Helmholtz H. Handbuch der physiologischen Optik. Leipzig: Leopold Voss; 1867

Helmholtz H. Versuch, das psychophysische Gesetz auf die Farbunterschiede trichromatischer Augen anzuwenden. Z Psychol Physiol Sinnesorg 1892; 3: 1–20

Hering E. Zur Lehre vom Lichtsinn. Vienna: Akad Wiss, Mathemat-Naturwiss; 1874: 169–204

Jacobs GH. Color vision. Annu Rev Psychol 1976; 27: 63–89

Kalmus H. The familial distribution of congenital tritanopia with some remarks on similar conditions. Ann Hum Genet 1955; 20: 39–56

Krastel H. Farbsinn. In: W Straub, P Kroll, HJ Küchle, eds. Augenärztliche Untersuchungsmethoden. 2. Auflage. Stuttgart: Enke Verlag; 1995: 537–566

Krastel H. Farbensinnprüfung in der Praxis. Klin Monatsbl Augenheilkd 2007; 224: 29–56

Krastel H, Kolling G, Schiefer U, et al. Qualitätsanforderungen an die Untersuchung des Farbsinns. Ophthalmologe 2009; 106: 1083–1102

Kries JA. Über Farbensysteme. Z Psychol Physiol Sinnesorg 1897; 13: 241–324

Lanthony P. Color vision. Annee Ther Clin Ophtalmol 1987; 38: 117–133

Lennie P, D'Zmura M. Mechanisms of color vision. Crit Rev Neurobiol 1988; 3: 333–400

Michael CR. Color vision. N Engl J Med 1973; 288: 724–728

Nathans J. The evolution and physiology of human color vision: insights from molecular genetic studies of visual pigments. Neuron 1999; 24: 299–312

Ripps H, Weale RA. Color vision. Annu Rev Psychol 1969; 20: 193–216

Swanson WH, Cohen JM. Color vision. Ophthalmol Clin North Am 2003; 16: 179–203

Volk D, Fry GA. Effect of quality of illumination and distance of observation upon performance in the Ishihara test. Am J Optom Arch Am Acad Optom 1947; 24: 99–122

Walraven PL. Color vision. Annu Rev Psychol 1972; 23: 347–374

Weitz CJ, Miyake Y, Shinzato K, et al. Human tritanopia associated with two amino acid substitutions in the blue-sensitive opsin. Am J Hum Genet 1992a; 50: 498–507

Weitz CJ, Went LN, Nathans J. Human tritanopia associated with a third amino acid substitution in the blue-sensitive visual pigment. Am J Hum Genet 1992a; 51: 444–446

Welsch N, Liebmann C. Farben: Natur, Technik, Kunst. Heidelberg, Berlin: Spektrum Akademischer Verlag; 2003

Young T. On the theory of light and colour. Phil Trans Roy Soc 1802; 20–71

Zrenner E. Farbsinnprüfungen: Grundlagen, Meßverfahren und Anwendungen bei angeborenen und erworbenen Farbsinnstörungen. In: OE Lund, TN Waubke, eds. Augenerkrankungen im Kindesalter. Stuttgart: Enke; 1985: 263–286

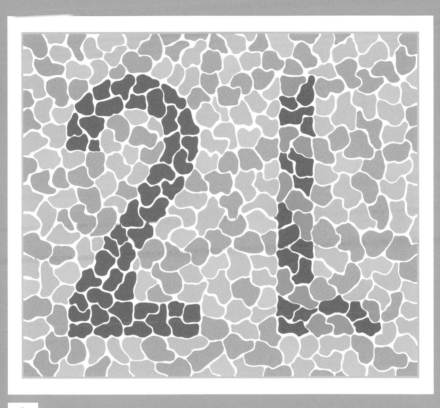

L

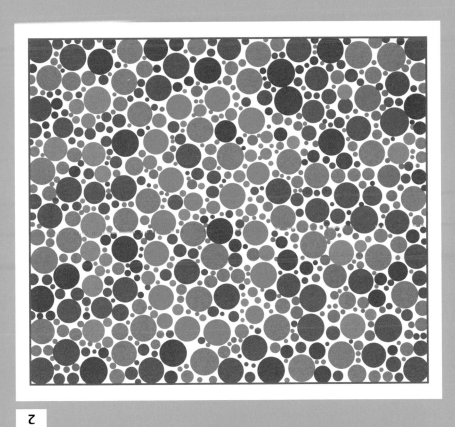

2

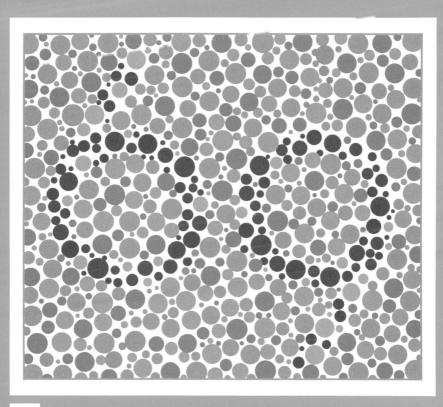

3

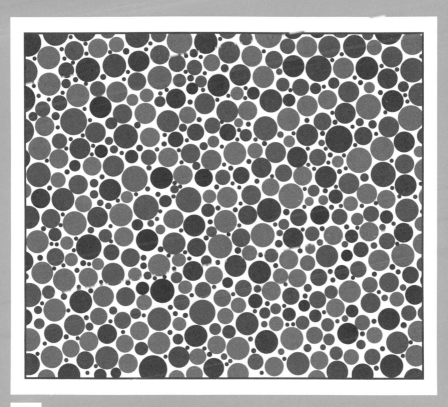

4

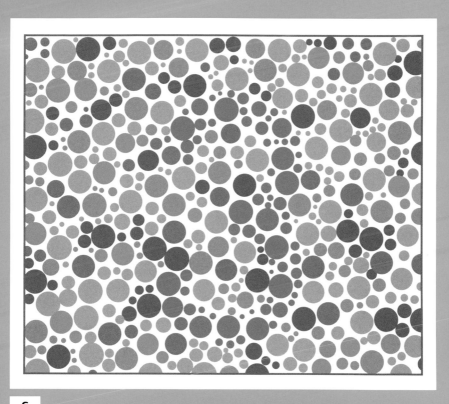

5

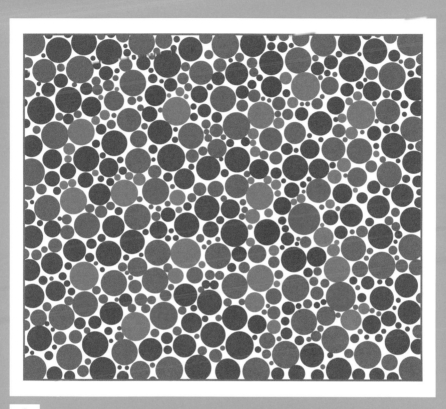

9

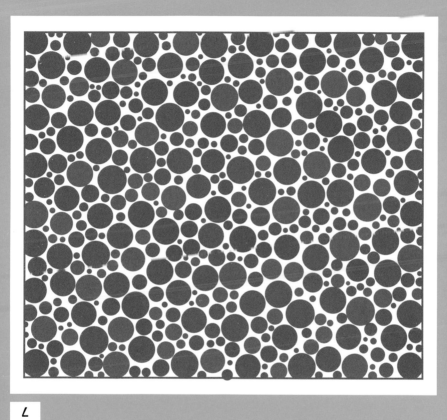

7

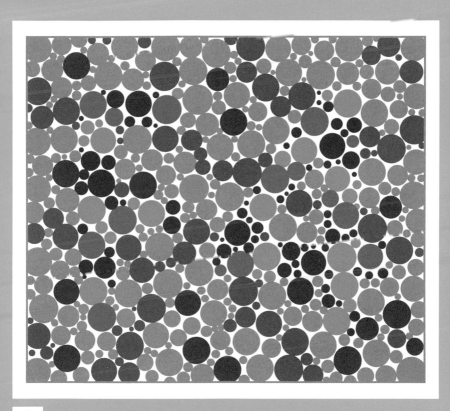

8

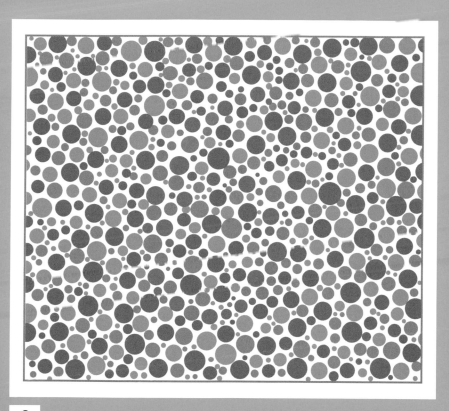

6

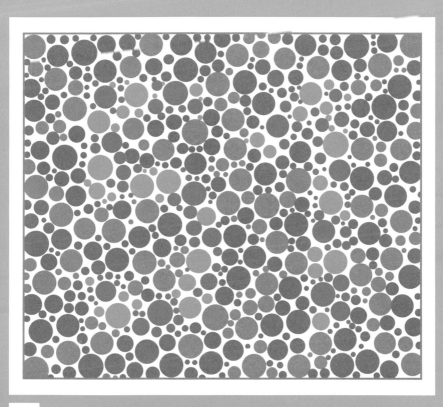

10

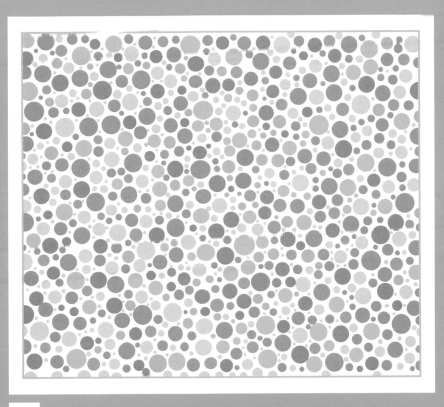

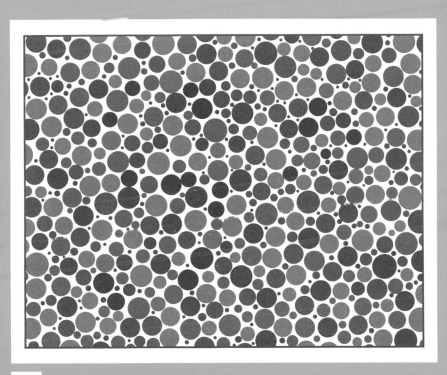

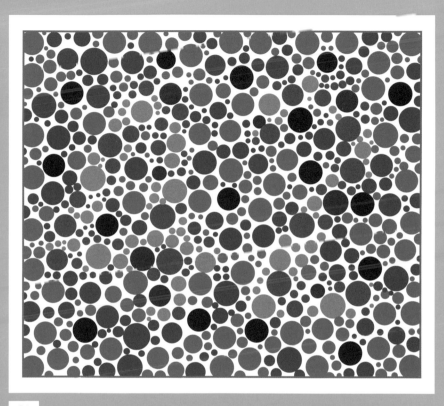

13

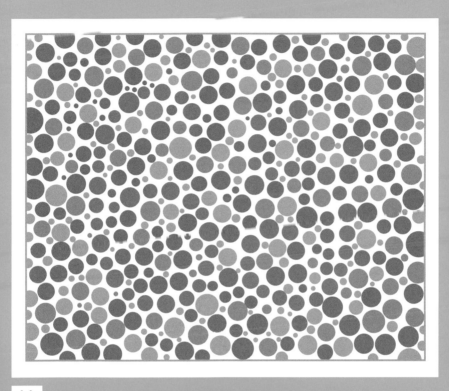

14

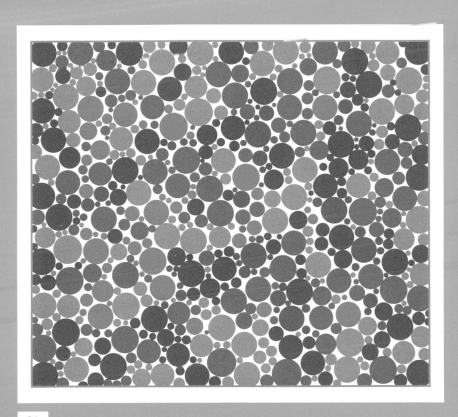

15

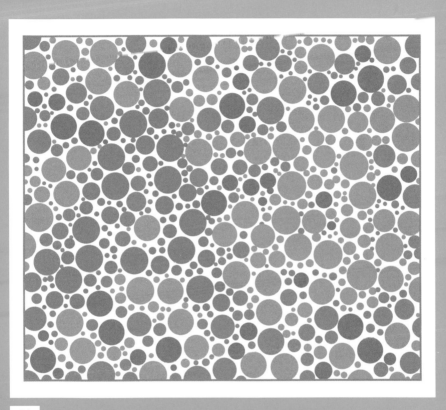

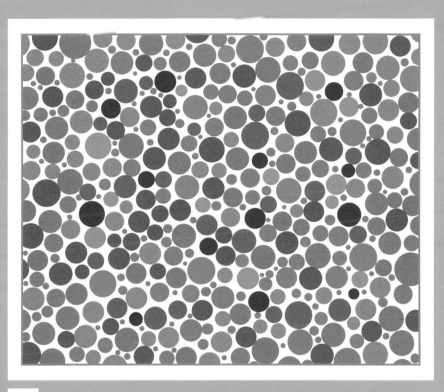

17

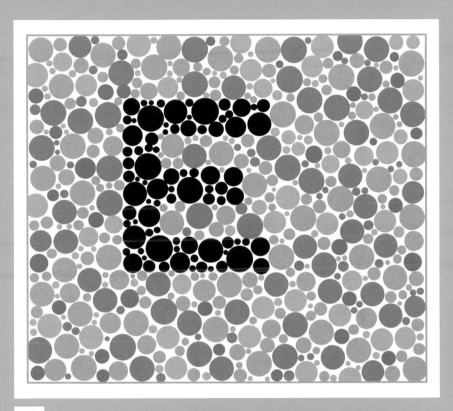

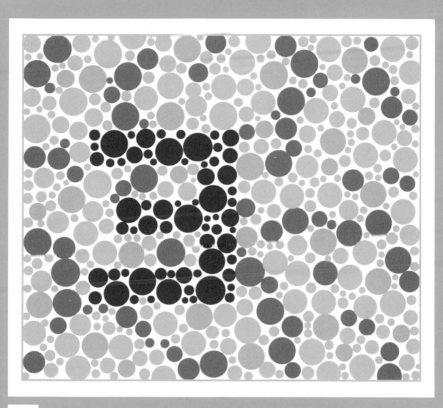

19

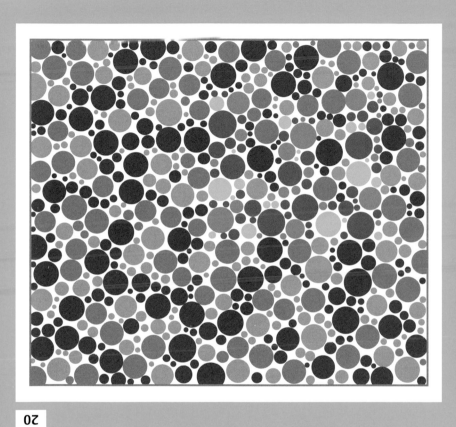

20

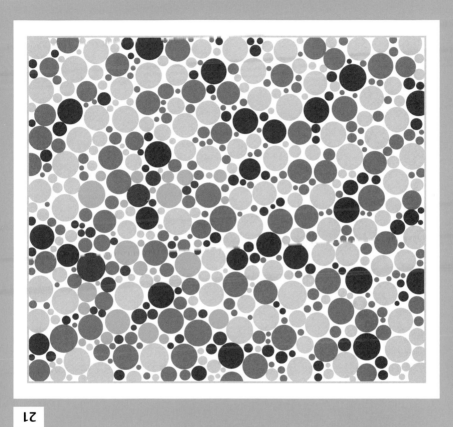

21

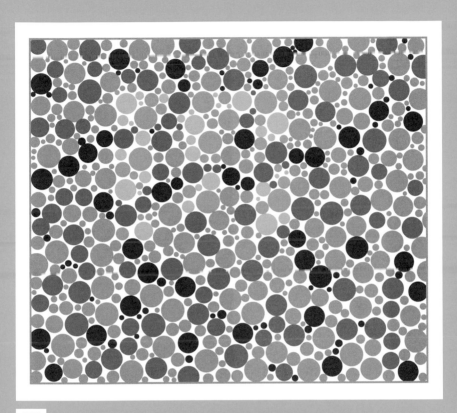

22

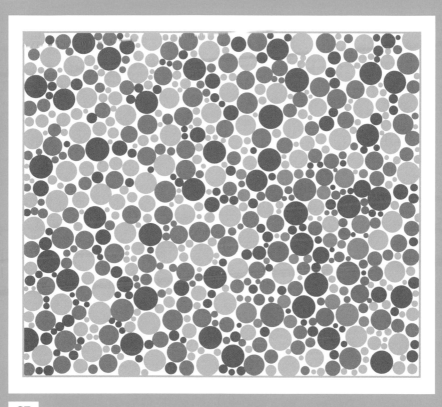

23

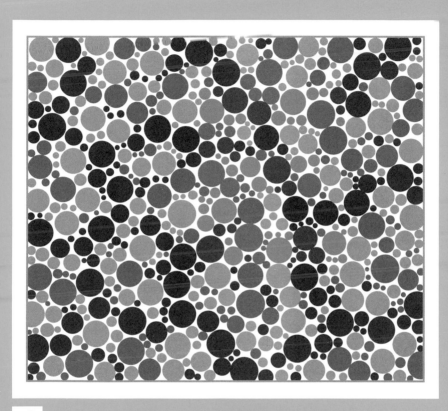

24

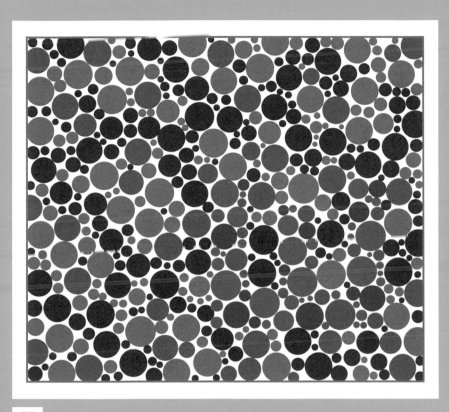

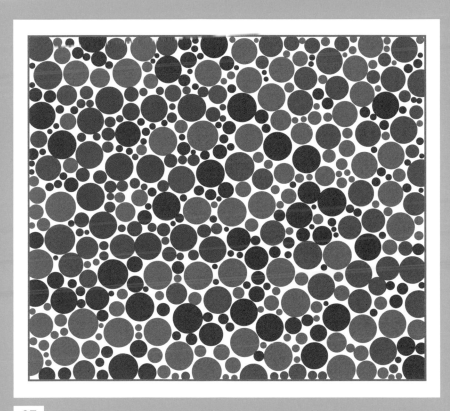

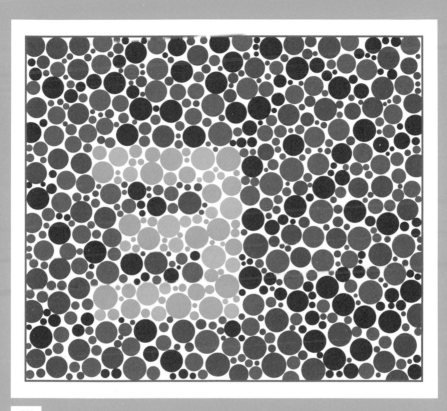

27

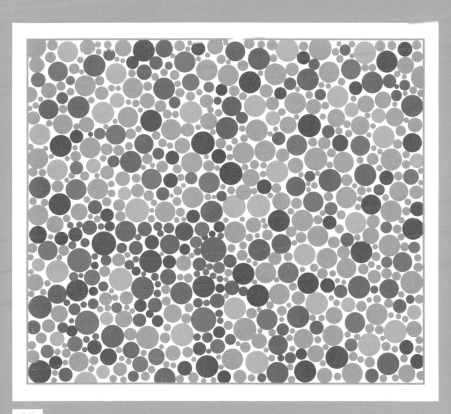

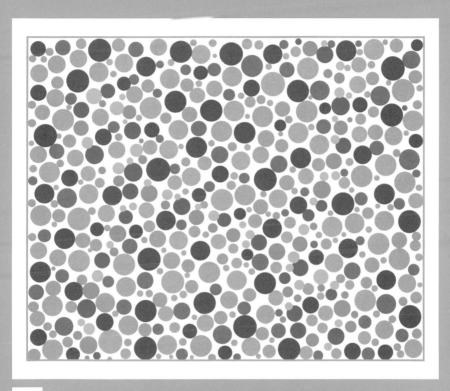

29

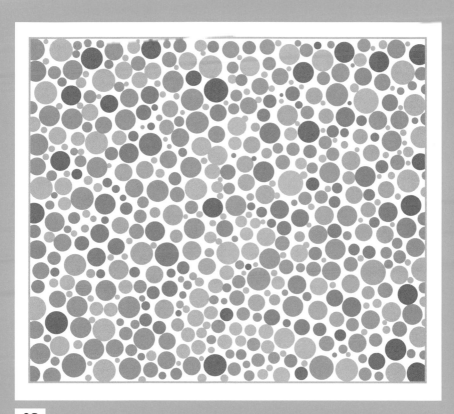

30

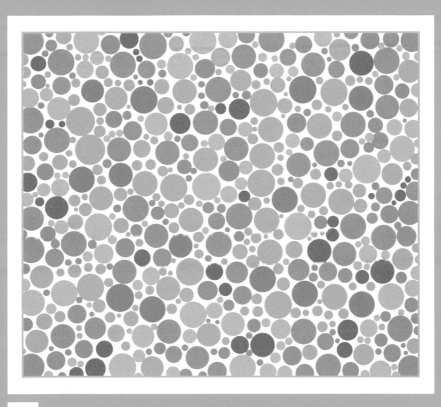

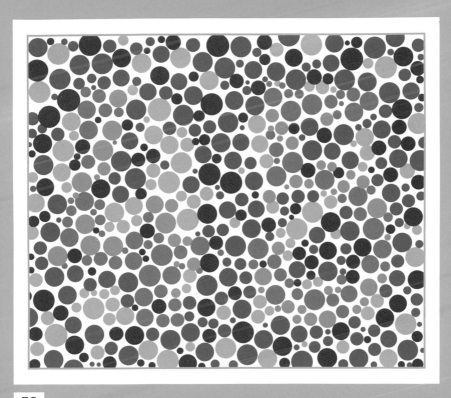